E ANDERSON, A
Anderson, AnnMarie
Meet a dentist!

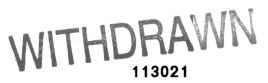

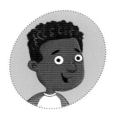
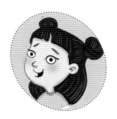

In Our Neighborhood

Meet a Dentist!

by AnnMarie Anderson

Illustrations by Lisa Hunt

Children's Press®
An imprint of Scholastic Inc.

SCHOLASTIC

Special thanks to our content consultants:

Monica Ashok, D.D.S.   Jeffrey Pivor, D.D.S.
Brooklyn, NY   Norwalk, CT

Library of Congress Cataloging-in-Publication Data
Names: Anderson, AnnMarie, author. | Hunt, Lisa, 1973– illustrator.
Title: In our neighborhood. Meet a dentist!/AnnMarie Anderson; illustrations by Lisa Hunt.
Other titles: Meet a dentist
Description: First edition. | New York: Children's Press, an imprint of Scholastic Inc., 2021. | Series: In our
  neighborhood | Includes index. | Audience: Ages 5–7. | Audience: Grades K–1. | Summary: "This book
  introduces the role of dentists in their community"— Provided by publisher.
Identifiers: LCCN 2021058745 (print) | LCCN 2021058746 (ebook) | ISBN 9781338769005 (library binding) |
  ISBN 9781338769067 (paperback) | ISBN 9781338769098 (ebook)
Subjects: LCSH: Dentists—Juvenile literature. | Dentistry—Juvenile literature.
Classification: LCC RK63 .A533 2021 (print) | LCC RK63 (ebook) | DDC 617.6092—dc23
LC record available at https://lccn.loc.gov/2021058745
LC ebook record available at https://lccn.loc.gov/2021058746

10 9 8 7 6 5 4 3 2 1   22 23 24 25 26

Printed in Heshan, China 62
First edition, 2022

Series produced by Spooky Cheetah Press
Prototype design by Maria Bergós/Book & Look
Page design by Kathleen Petelinsek/The Design Lab

Photos ©: 7: Anne-Sophie Bost/age fotostock; 12 left: Monkey Business
Images Ltd/age fotostock; 13 left: Photography/John Birdsall/age fotostock;
13 right: Airman 1st Class Kaylee Dubois/PJF Military Collection/Alamy
Images; 15: John Coletti/Getty Images; 17: tim gartside/Alamy Images; 18:
andresr/Getty Images; 25: Yarinca/Getty Images; 31 top left: Vasyl Rogan/
Dreamstime.

All other photos © Shutterstock.

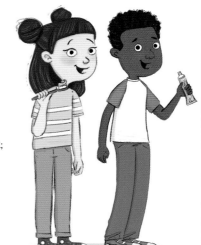

Table of Contents

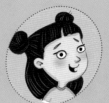

OUR NEIGHBORHOOD

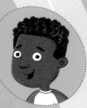

Hi! I'm Emma. This is my best friend, Theo. Welcome to our neighborhood!

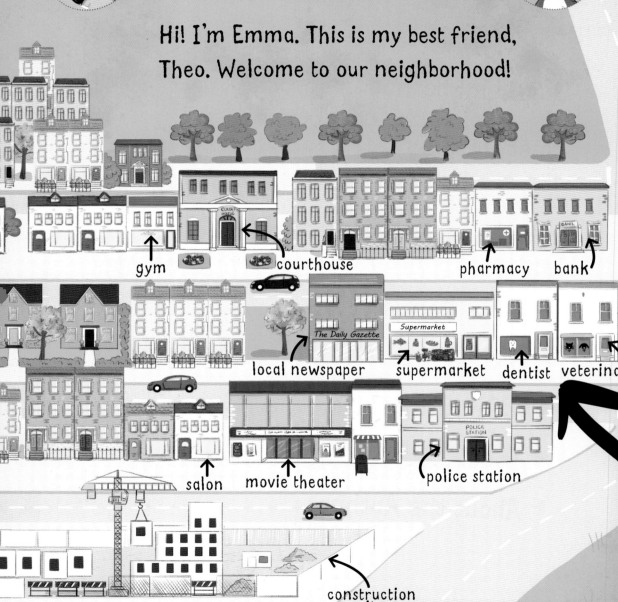

gym

courthouse

pharmacy

bank

The Daily Gazette

local newspaper

Supermarket

supermarket

dentist

veterina

salon

movie theater

POLICE STATION

police station

construction site

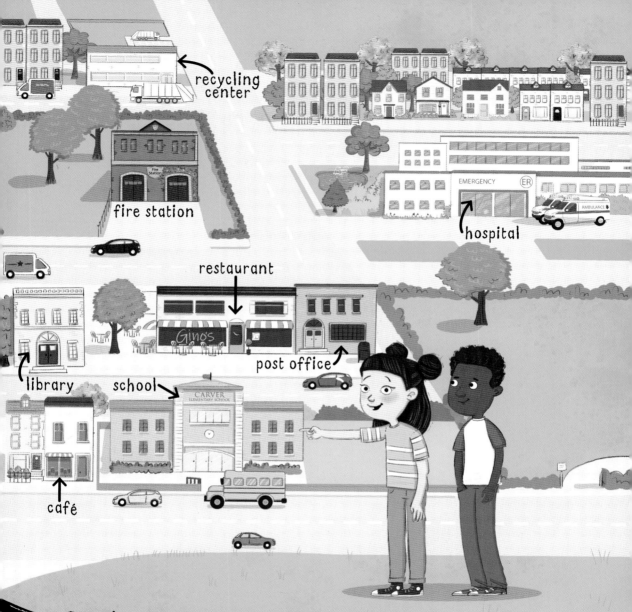

recycling center

fire station

hospital

EMERGENCY ER

AMBULANCE

restaurant

Gino's

post office

library

school

CARVER ELEMENTARY SCHOOL

café

Our dentist, Dr. Suárez, has her office over there. One day Dr. Suárez visited our class in school. She talked to us about how to keep our teeth healthy.

The day before Dr. Suárez came in, we started a science experiment. Our teacher, Mr. Garcia, gave each table an egg. We put the eggs in jars and covered them with cola.

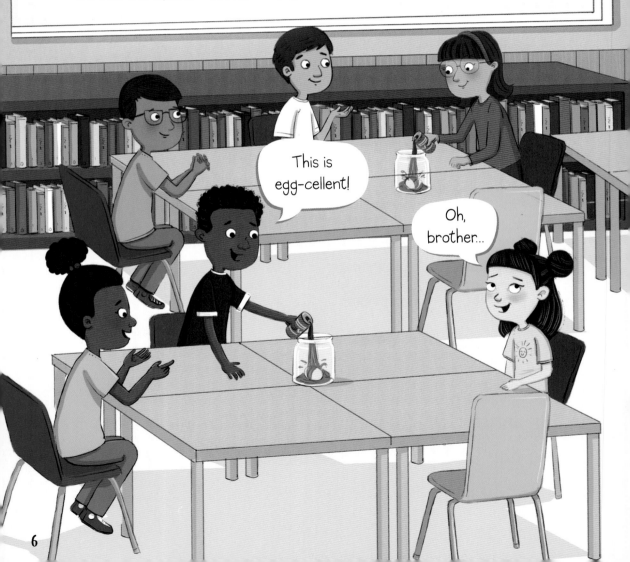

This is egg-cellent!

Oh, brother...

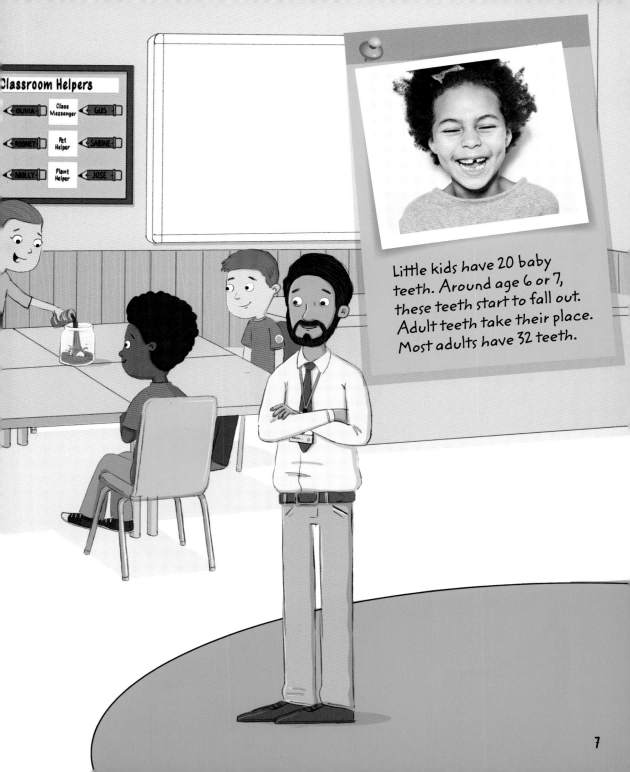

Little kids have 20 baby teeth. Around age 6 or 7, these teeth start to fall out. Adult teeth take their place. Most adults have 32 teeth.

MEET DR. SUÁREZ

The next day, when Dr. Suárez arrived, we took our eggs out of the cola. They had turned dark brown! Mr. Garcia gave us toothbrushes and toothpaste. When we brushed the eggs, they turned white again.

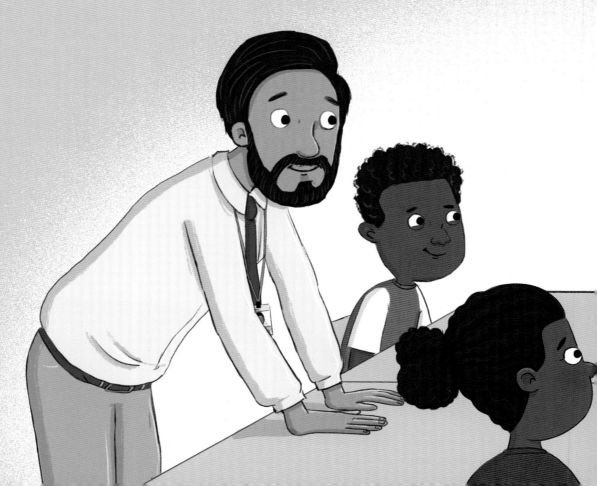

Dr. Suárez said that the eggshell was like the surface of our teeth. The egg was brown because some cola was left behind after we took it out of the jar. The same thing happens when we eat. Plaque is left behind on our teeth.

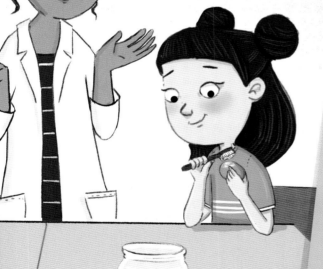

That is why flossing and brushing are so important!

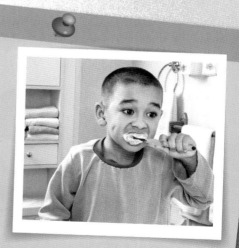

Plaque is a sticky film that contains bacteria and coats your teeth. Flossing and brushing help get rid of plaque between and on your teeth.

9

"We have bacteria in our mouth," Dr. Suárez explained. "That bacteria turns the food that's left on our teeth into acid. The acid can make small holes, or cavities, in our teeth."

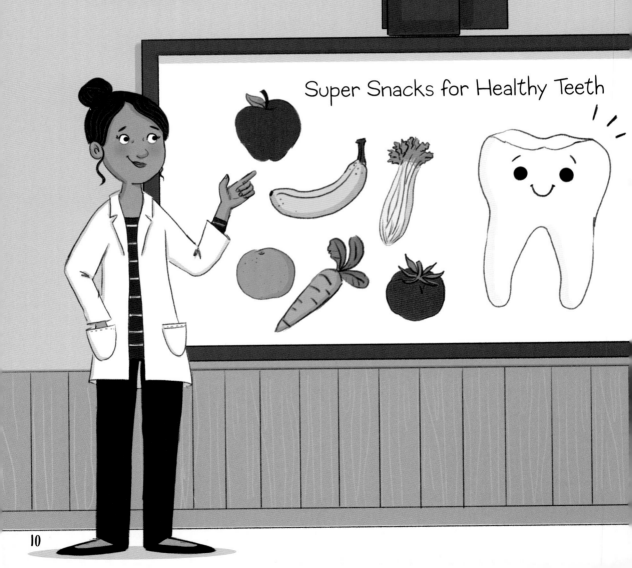

Super Snacks for Healthy Teeth

Dr. Suárez said that food and drinks like candy and soda have a lot of sugar that sticks to teeth. That's why it's best to eat them only sometimes.

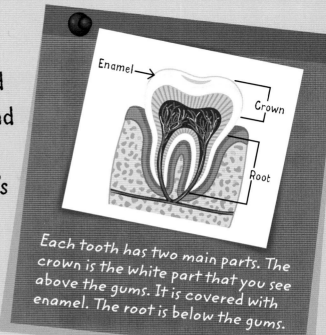

Enamel → | Crown

Root

Each tooth has two main parts. The crown is the white part that you see above the gums. It is covered with enamel. The root is below the gums.

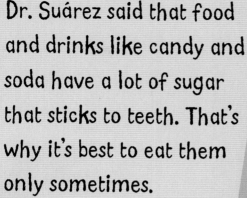

I'm glad I brought apple slices for snack today!

My dad packed carrot sticks.

After her presentation, Dr. Suárez told us about different types of dentists.

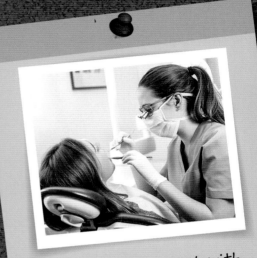

General dentists work with patients of all ages. They provide all dental care, including teaching their patients how to keep their teeth healthy.

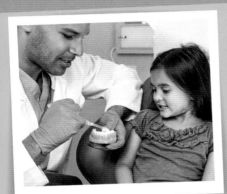

Pediatric dentists care for infants, children, and teens. They help their patients keep their teeth, gums, and mouths healthy.

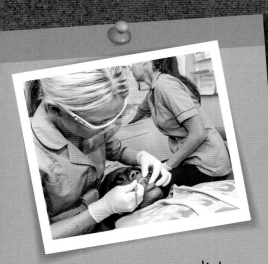

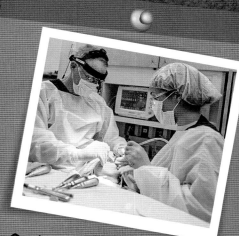

Orthodontists are specialists. They straighten crooked teeth, which helps people chew better and gives them a nice smile.

Oral surgeons remove teeth. They also perform surgeries and other procedures on patients' jaws and gums.

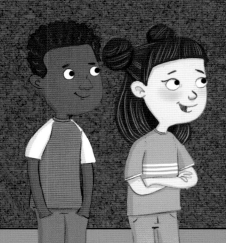

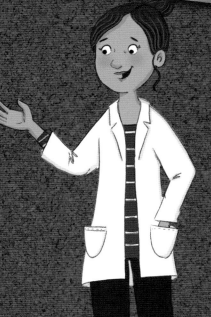

Then Dr. Suárez had to go back to work. Theo and I would see her after school, though. We both had appointments for our cleanings and checkups.

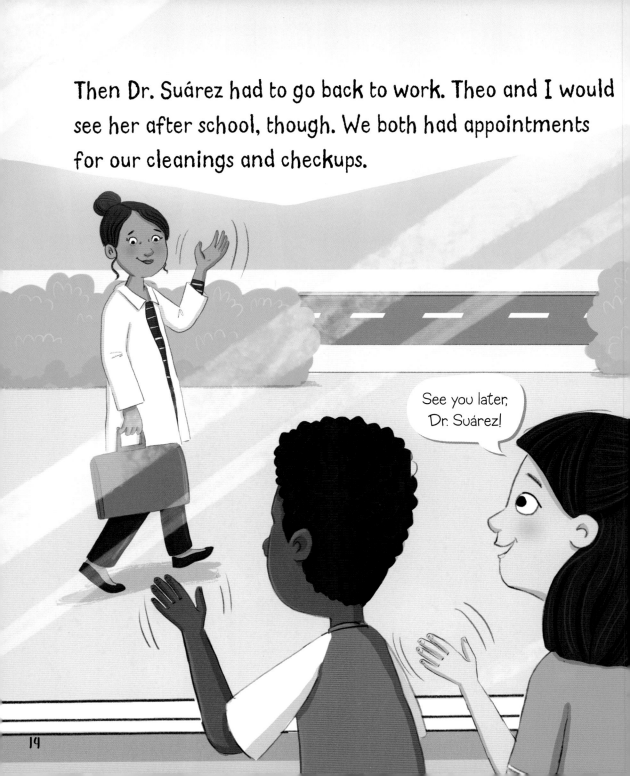

See you later, Dr. Suárez!

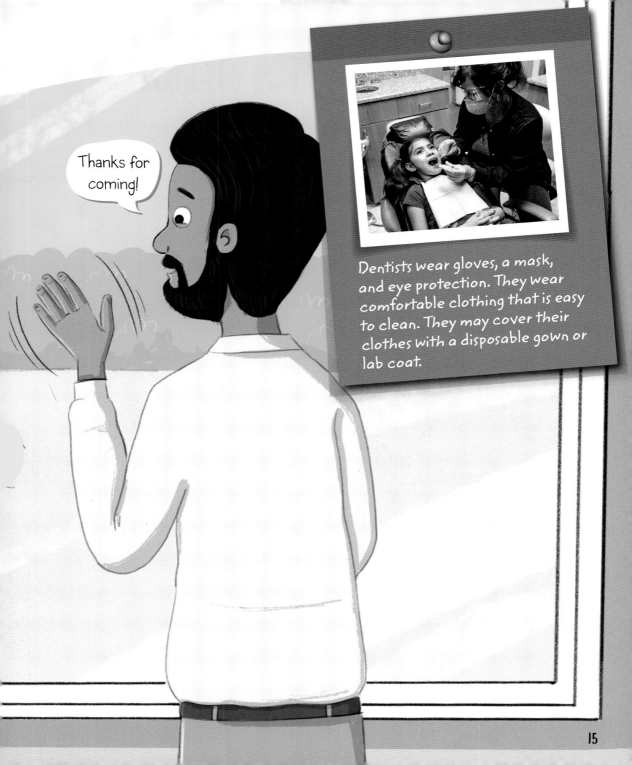

Thanks for coming!

Dentists wear gloves, a mask, and eye protection. They wear comfortable clothing that is easy to clean. They may cover their clothes with a disposable gown or lab coat.

AT THE DENTIST'S OFFICE

When I got to Dr. Suárez's office later that day, Theo was already in the waiting room. After a few minutes, Mark, the dental hygienist, came to get me.

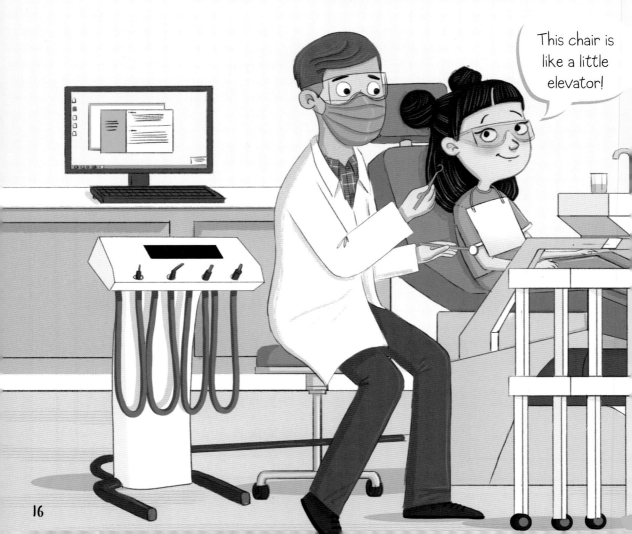

This chair is like a little elevator!

Mark showed me to a big chair. He raised the chair up so he could see my teeth. There was a big, bright light over my head. Mark gave me sunglasses to wear. Then he used special tools to clean my teeth.

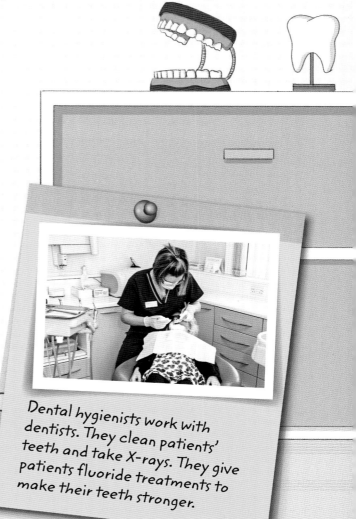

Dental hygienists work with dentists. They clean patients' teeth and take X-rays. They give patients fluoride treatments to make their teeth stronger.

Mark took X-rays of my mouth.

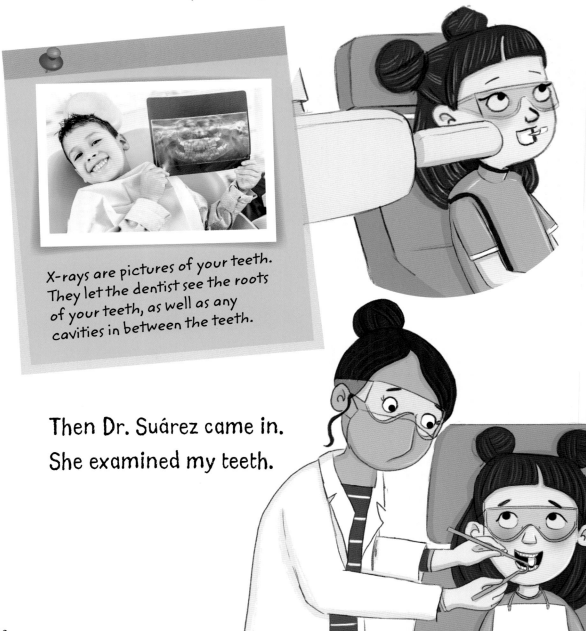

X-rays are pictures of your teeth. They let the dentist see the roots of your teeth, as well as any cavities in between the teeth.

Then Dr. Suárez came in.
She examined my teeth.

After that, she showed me my X-rays and told me I had a small cavity. I would have to get a filling.

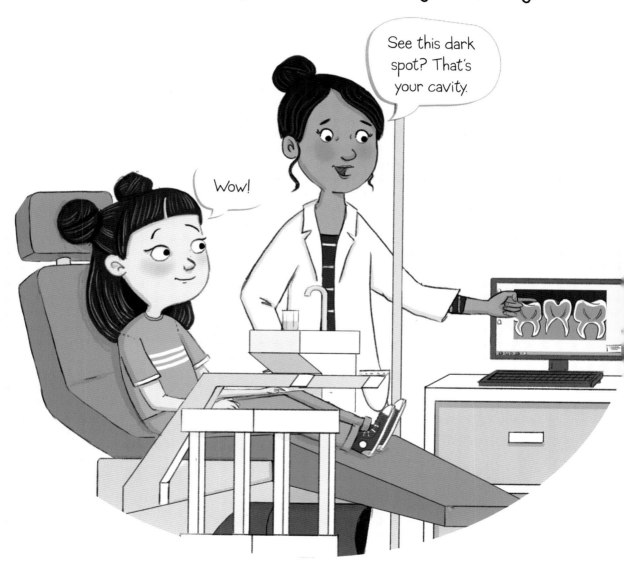

Then it was Theo's turn. Dr. Suárez told him his six-year molars had come in. These teeth come in at the back of the mouth when a person is six or seven years old. Unlike other teeth, molars don't replace baby teeth.

Molars are permanent teeth—so you need to take good care of them!

Dr. Suárez told Theo his molars had deep grooves. She would paint a coating, or sealant, on his molars to protect them from getting cavities.

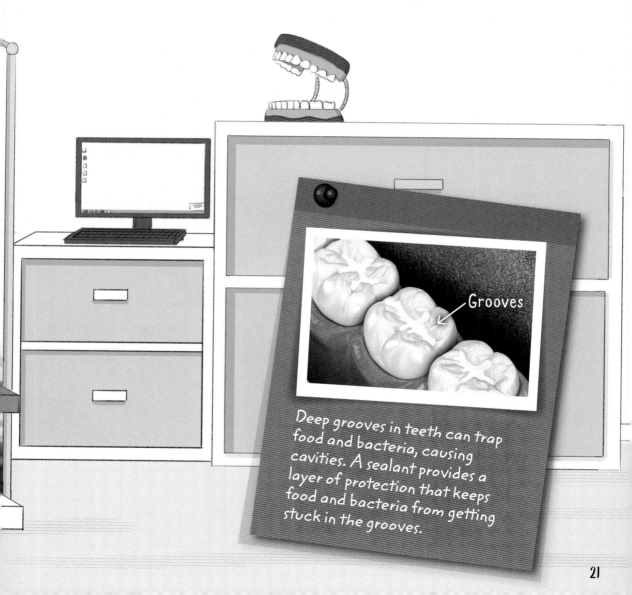

Grooves

Deep grooves in teeth can trap food and bacteria, causing cavities. A sealant provides a layer of protection that keeps food and bacteria from getting stuck in the grooves.

GETTING A FILLING

The following Saturday, I went back to Dr. Suárez's office to have my cavity filled.

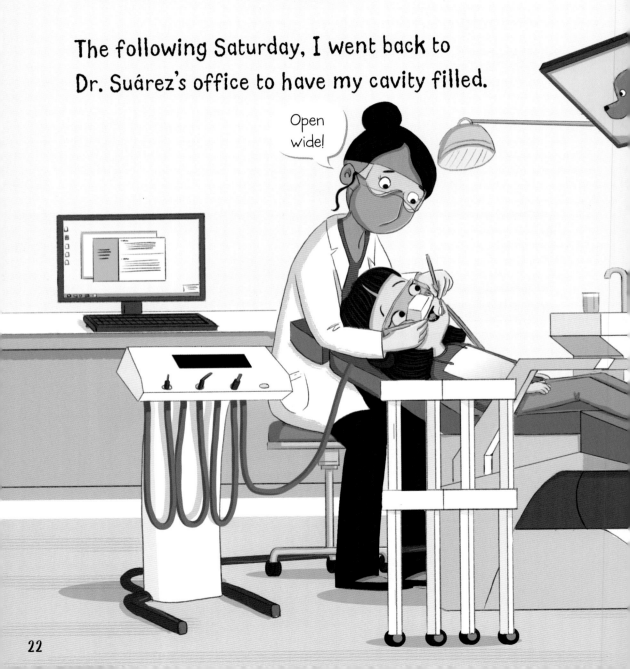

First Dr. Suárez put a small mask over my nose. She asked me to breathe in and out slowly. She cleaned out the cavity in my tooth and filled the hole. I got to watch TV while she worked!

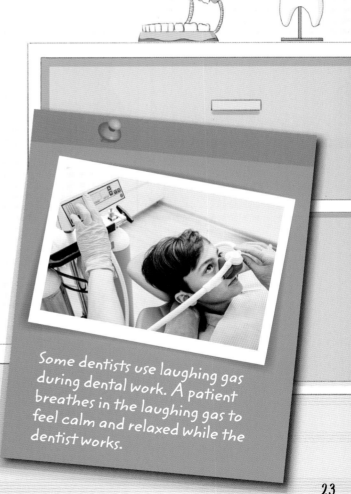

Some dentists use laughing gas during dental work. A patient breathes in the laughing gas to feel calm and relaxed while the dentist works.

After my cavity was filled, I left Dr. Suárez's office with a toothbrush, toothpaste, dental floss, a book, and a sticker!

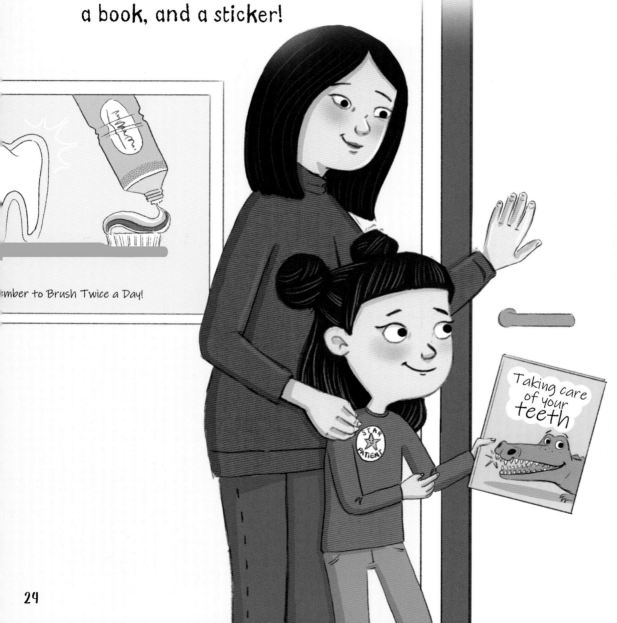

mber to Brush Twice a Day!

Taking care of your teeth

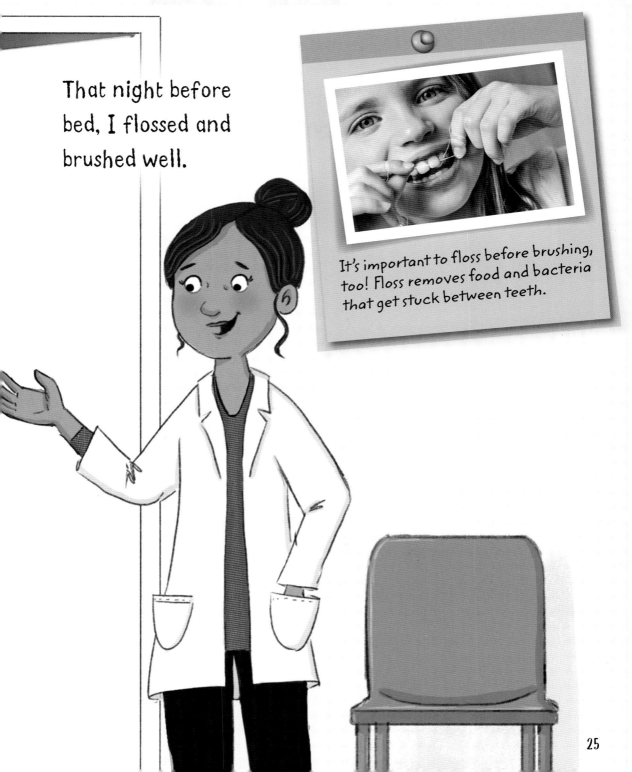

That night before bed, I flossed and brushed well.

It's important to floss before brushing, too! Floss removes food and bacteria that get stuck between teeth.

Six months later, Theo and I saw Dr. Suárez for another checkup. She gave us both great news— no new cavities!

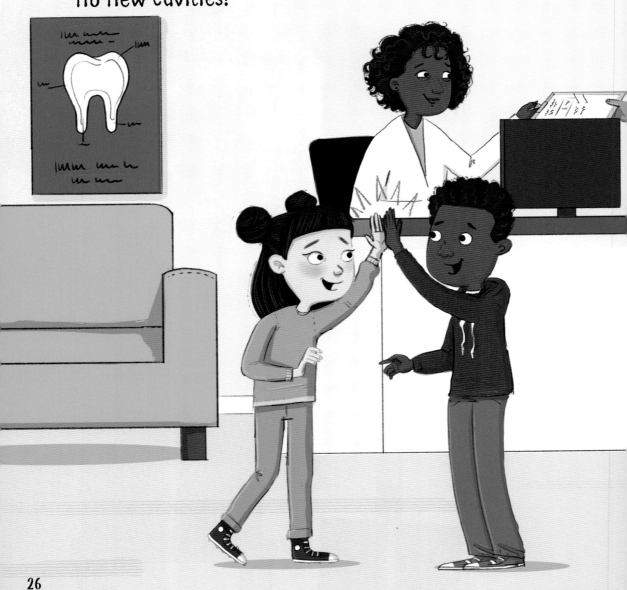

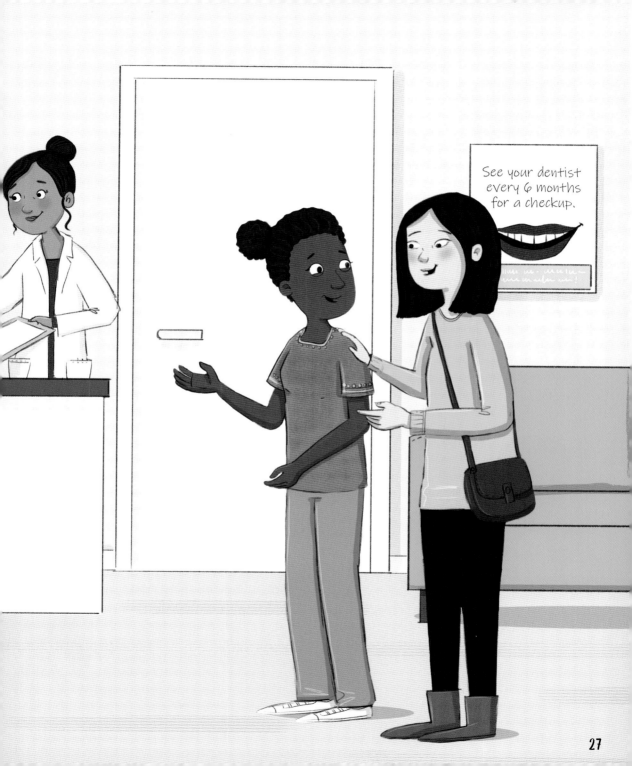

See your dentist every 6 months for a checkup.

27

Ask a Dentist

Theo asked Dr. Suárez some questions about her job.

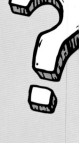
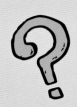

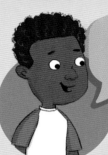

How many years did you train to become a pediatric dentist?

I attended four years of dental school. Then I spent two years working in a dental hospital just with kids.

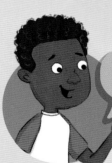

What is the best thing about your job?

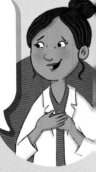

I love my job! I really enjoy working with families. I like teaching good habits that I hope will stay with them for the rest of their lives.

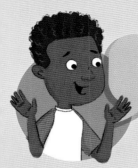

Why are baby teeth so important even though they fall out?

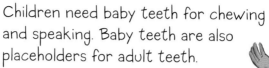

Children need baby teeth for chewing and speaking. Baby teeth are also placeholders for adult teeth.

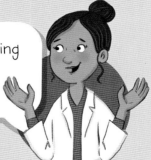

Have you ever had a cavity?

Yes. The first time I went to the dentist as a kid, I had four cavities! But I haven't had one since because I floss and brush every morning and evening!

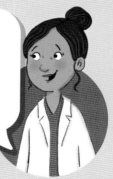

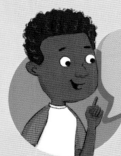

What is one thing most people don't know about being a dentist?

Dentists have to go through a lot of medical training before they become doctors.

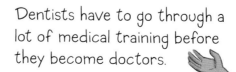

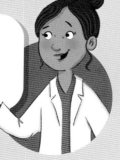

Dr. Suárez's Tips for Taking Great Care of Your Teeth

- Make sure to floss at least once a day before brushing.

- Be sure to brush your teeth at least twice a day—in the morning and before bed.

- Brush for at least two minutes each time!

- Limit sweet foods and drinks.

- Visit your dentist twice a year for a cleaning and checkup.

A Dentist's Tools

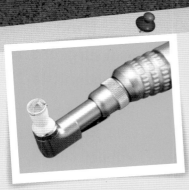

Rubber cup polisher:
Dentists and hygienists use polishers to clean stains and plaque from teeth.

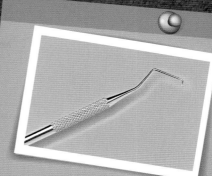

Scaler: Dentists and hygienists use a scaler to remove plaque from the teeth and gumline.

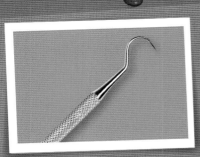

Explorer tool: Dentists use this metal tool with a small point at the end to check for cavities.

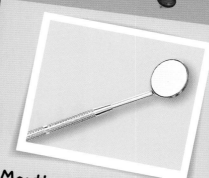

Mouth mirror: Dentists use a mouth mirror to look at parts of the mouth that are hard to see.

Index

About the Author

AnnMarie Anderson has written numerous books for young readers—from easy readers to novels. She lives in Brooklyn, New York, with her husband and two sons. She loves minty-flavored toothpaste!